WOMB *to* HARVARD

300 DAYS SECRET OF GOD AVATARS

ISBN : 978-93-95266-39-0 (Paperback)

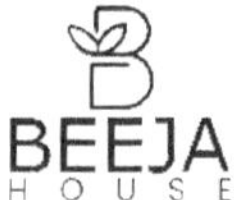

Published by: Beeja House

First Printing Edition 2023
Printed By: Repro Books Limited

Author Email: smanoharmalu@gmail.com

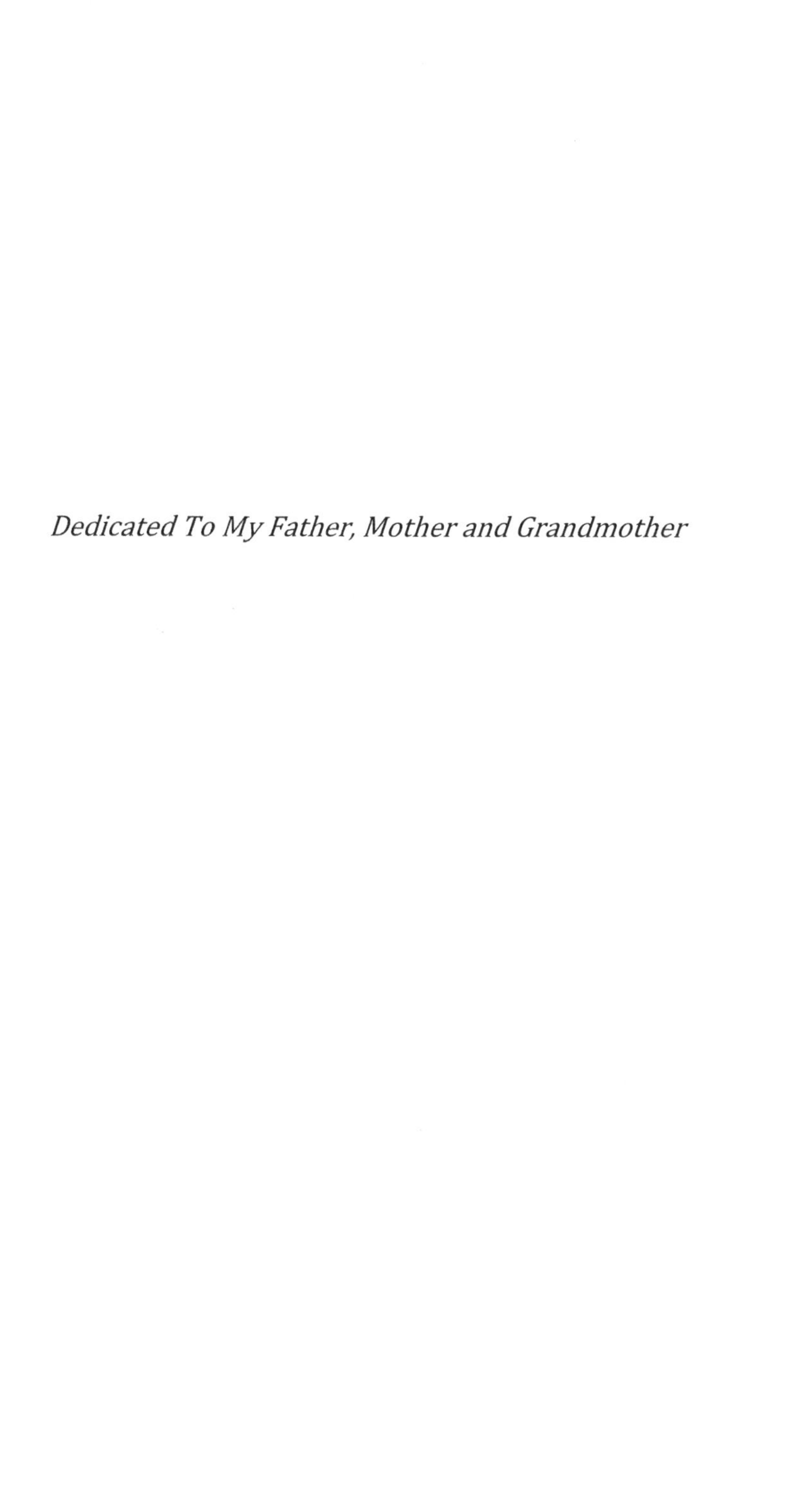

Dedicated To My Father, Mother and Grandmother

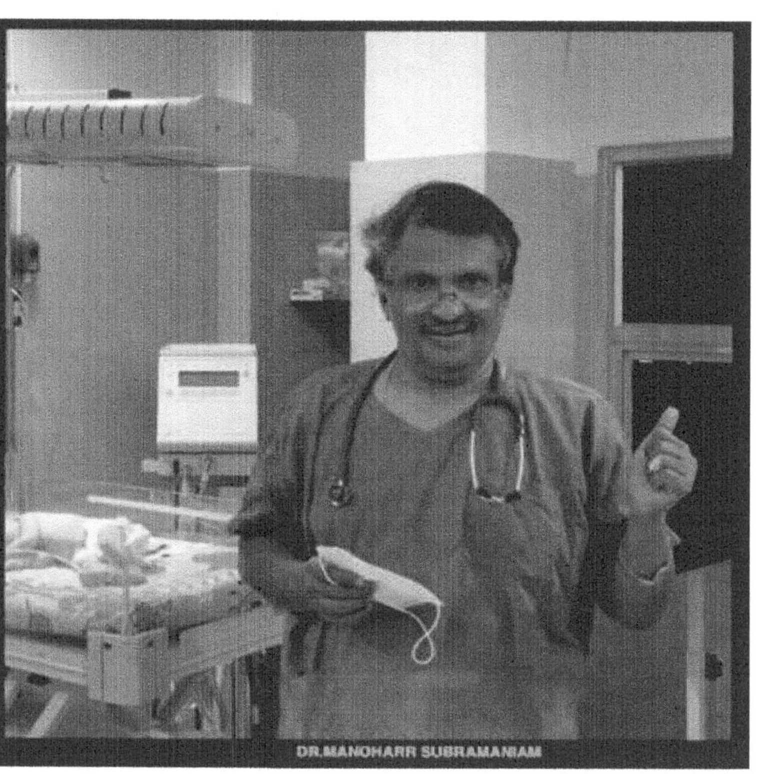
DR.MANOHARR SUBRAMANIAM

About The Author

Dr Manohar Subramaniam has 25 years of experience in neonatology & paediatrics, now a consultant at Rajendra hospital, Calicut.

This is not a medical book, it's for father and mother, and no medical jargon is used.

He says, "I am here as a mother-baby parental coach with a mission to help a million mothers to have their desired kids through the womb to Harvard hub. "

Every mother desire to have super healthy, sensitive, intelligent smart babies who can love humanity and face the challenges of the new world, and technology and contribute to the same for a better

It can only happen when mothers are empowered with knowledge of how to guide their babies from "Womb to Harvard or Oxford or IIM, AIIMS, or IAS, IPS or IIT …. it has to start from the womb and before starting from conceiving smartly in the womb, the journey of entering motherhood begins with being a wife, children to childhood starts with a baby father-to-fatherhood starts with a husband all hoods start from marriage to conception. All these hoods have great procreation of self, the base and foundation starting from marriage to conception.

For the last 25 years, he is a very successful, busy newborn & child specialist.

People approve of him because he treats their kids with love and affection.

He made my parents understand the lifestyle they should follow for the benefit and have smart babies they dreamt of in a language they understand without medical jargon.

One should use language that can help in initiating a healthy conversation in order to connect with the unborn.

Through this journey, he hopes that readers will get to experience a whole lot of engaging ideas of healthy parenting. Wishing you all the best and for your babies, have your baby gene expressed the way you want.

From conception till 3 years of age, give your child the best chance to cope with success with a customized plan for their life, learn more about our personalised development plan and how it works.

Help your little one reach their full potential with Womb to Harvard university.

Now, let the author start with what made him write this book.

Preface

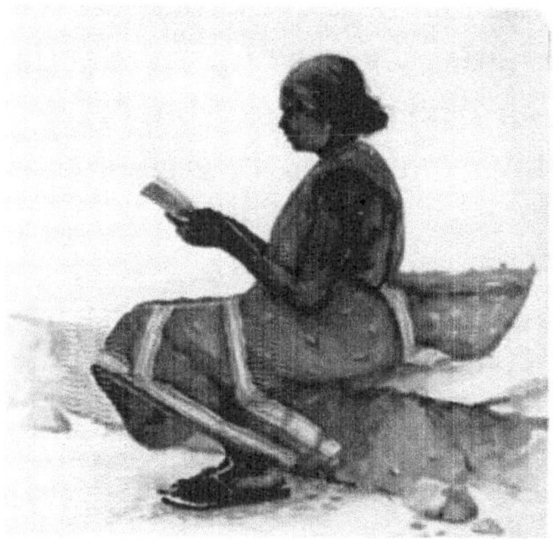

This is a well-researched book and created content in two sections.

The 1st section includes stories based on true events.

The 2nd section elaborates on tools: and different aspects of the stories.

A child's potential to become a genius is greatly influenced by the kind of intelligent/positive input they receive from their parents. Every parent hope that their child grows up to be successful, healthy, and a bright member of society.

They have no idea of how to get there or when they should start playing the role of a parent .. Only a small percentage of parents can fulfil their dream of sending their children to the best schools, tuitions, and universities by making substantial financial contributions and paying exorbitant fees. A delay in parental involvement is referred to as "delayed parenting".

Investing in womb university is the "process of pregnancy".

Invest in 1090 days to change the gene expression to your desired expression.

Pre-conception/ Conception/ Womb care & Nurturing / Natal & Postnatal care

Get the best out of motherhood from sparkle motherhood/ womb: the knowledge motherhood/ nutrition protection motherhood/personality motherhood to achieve motherhood.

An unborn child's brain produces 250,000 new cells every minute, allowing for rapid development during pregnancy.

He/she benefited physically, mentally, spiritually, and emotionally through mother's caregiving.

We hope that by educating mothers about the importance of prenatal care, we can help them bring forth babies who are healthy, intelligent, and creative thinkers.

Now is the time to lay the groundwork for what lies beneath the surface...

The real strength of a tree is in its unseen roots, which allow it to weather storms, extreme temperatures, and other terrifying forces of nature. Similarly, a human being's unseen roots are formed during preconception, conception, womb care and postnatal care.

 I have written this book and am excited to share strategies with you.

Contents

Section 1 1

300 Day Secret of Avatars 3

Soul Seeding 7

Implicit Memory (Unconscious Memory) 9

Spiritual-Gold-Plating or Galvanoplasty................11

Significance of a Father...13

True Story... Why? 15

True Story..19

    The Beginning of a Legacy 21

    Wonders Happen... 24

    Amma's Decision 32

    The Transformation... 39

    Happy Events & Dr. Thambi.............................. 46

    Analysis & Conclusion....................................... 50

Section 2 55

Preface 57

Epigenetics 63

    What Is Epigenetics? 64

    Role Of Epigenetic In Unborn Baby................... 65

    Prenatal Diet.. 65

    Pregnancy Exercise 66

    Pregnancy Hormone Prolactin 66

    Thyroid Hormones:.. 67

    Oestrogen: 67

Conclusion:..67

Progeny 68

(Generations Inheritance).......................................68

    The Key 69

    Theory Of Life In Force 70

Water and Spirituality 73

    Water in Ritual and Symbol.............................74

    Why is water important in Womb to Harvard Strategy?.....76

Motherhood..77

    Marriage 77

    Sparkle Mother: Lights the Next-Gen in Her Womb 79

    Womb Mother-300 Golden Days-Gods Own Secret.............81

Learning Inside The Womb 83

    Month 1 (1st Trimester) 89

    Month 3 (1st Trimester) 92

    Month 4 (2nd Trimester)..................................94

    Month 5 (2nd Trimester)..................................97

    Month 6 (2nd Trimester)..................................99

    Month 7 (3rd Trimester) 101

    Month 8 (3rd Trimester) 104

    Month 9 (3rd Trimester) 107

Birth!...110

    Baby's First Cry — Vagitus..............................110

Section 3 115

Coming Soon! 115

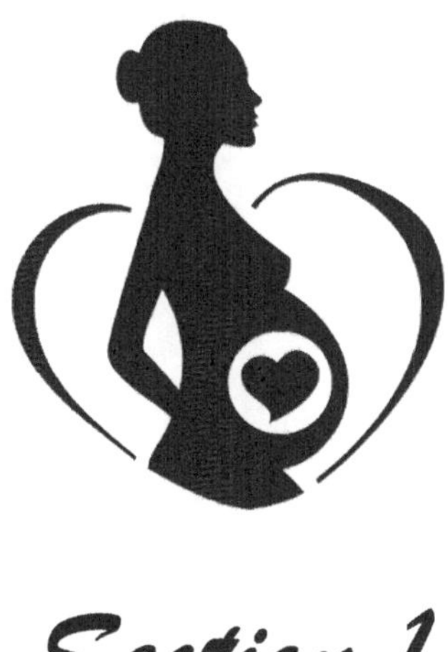

Section 1

Stories Shared are Based on True Life Stories

300 Day Secret of Avatars

Before I reveal the secret of CONCEPTION TO BIRTH CREATION OF AVATARS, 300-day secrets, 9 months period in "mother's womb". the foundation of mankind, even God needs these 300 days to create holy avatars.

Let me start with a real story that I witnessed in my life. I was working in a gulf country where they follow Shariya Law, I arrived from Ireland and on my first posting day, on the way to my posted hospital, I saw a huge crowd and a lot of policemen. I entered the hospital wherein they verified my ID and permitted me; I saw the Medical Officer In-charge and enquired what was happening, he said, "We will talk at lunch," I said, "Fine."

When I heard the story as a baby's doctor, naturally, I started thinking of my unborn and born baby.

The incident occurred 18 years back in a prestigious joint family where two brothers indulged in a quarrel related to a land dispute. The elder brother shot the younger brother. The younger brother's wife was pregnant, the elder brother was convicted and the judge read the final verdict. The judgement will be given by the unborn baby in the mother's womb after birth until he/she turns 18 years old. I landed on the day the boy delivered the judgement. What else could be the judgment? Mother nurturing and talking to him as Devakimata would have done to Lord Krishna.

This boy was lured with money and received a marriage opportunity from a pretty woman. He was not disturbed but he only spoke what his mother had nurtured and spoke to him in the womb. In Arabic, he said, "I want justice, he shot my father and he needs to be shot. The judgment of the boy was carried out."

How can the boy be lured?

The nurturing of a mother can never fail, though Lord Krishna was brought up in Ayodhya after being born, he did exactly what Devakimata had nurtured, requested to kill the evil king who murdered her 6 babies and to protect the land, he did what he was requested to as an unborn baby.

EVEN GOD NEED THESE 300 DAYS to create Avatars. A pregnant mother is an interface between the external world and the unborn. The first school for every man and woman is his/her mother's womb. The greatest teacher is the expectant mother.

Mythology is a witness to the womb expression, even holy avatars needed these 300 days of womb university. Almighty never said I will come and do it for you. He always had an avatar to represent himself as a holy avatar.

Krishna was born and nurtured by Devakimata in the womb with affirmations and love to be a saviour from Kansa and save humanity from evil, in India, it's also known as Garbha Vidya.

Even gene expression can be changed by using the 300-day secrets.

Prahlada carries genes of Rakshasa. The nurturing words of Naradha to the unborn Prahalad bloomed into a great Lord Vishnu also known as Bhakta Vatsal.

The following example sets proof of learning in the womb.
Unborn Abhimanyu heard Arjuna narrating to his mother how to break the Chakravayuha (Padmavayuha) in the womb and he did that in *Mahabharata*.

Every Avatar has to be born. Jesus took birth, and Prophet Muhammed took birth to save humanity. Similarly, Karthikeyan demolishes Asura, and Ayyappan demolishes Mahishi.

These innumerable pieces of evidence in mythology indicate that God needs a mother's womb for 300 days to create an avatar. That's why these 300 days are known as "300-DAY SECRETS OF GOD AVATARS".

300 days process involves the following:

- Soul Seedling
- Implicit Memory
- Spiritual-Gold-Plating or Galvanoplasty
- Significance of a Father

Soul Seeding

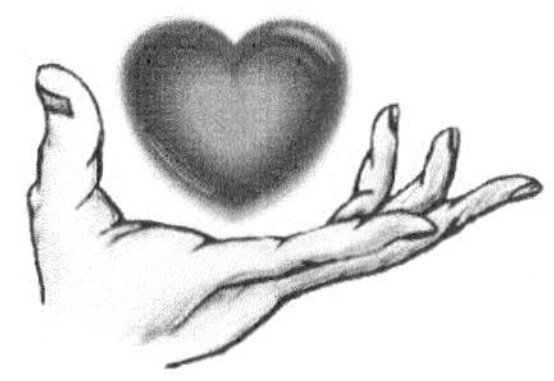

The umbilical cord not only carries oxygen, glucose, and other nutrients for growth and development but also carries the mother's emotions.

A mother should listen to a particular song regularly that she likes and enjoys. You will notice the movement in the womb whenever the mother listens to the song.

The "MOVEMENT" is the language of an unborn "COMMUNICATION".

The response of the baby will eventually be the same towards the song and as well to the voice of the mother. The mother should communicate with the child, and introduce herself as well as the other family members.

As the relationship between the mother and the unborn deepens, start "NURTURING" the mother specifically talks about skills and qualities the baby should have and dos & don'ts. The result is amazing. The mother sees a replica as desired by her in the unborn baby.

Practising these steps, the "soul seeding", "communication" and "nurturing" helps in personality development.

Implicit Memory (Unconscious Memory)

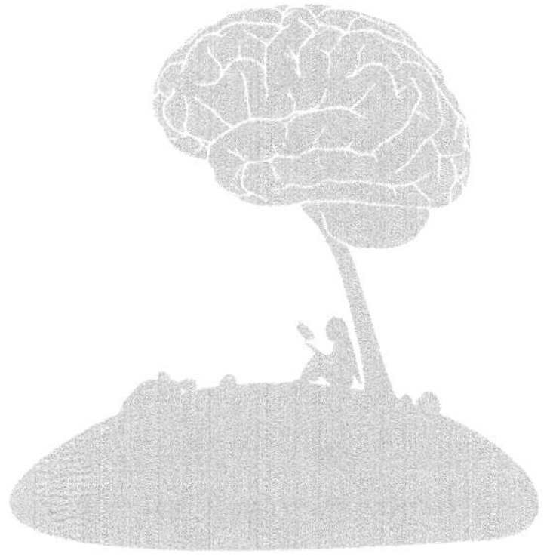

During 28 weeks of pregnancy, all the vital senses, vision, hearing, taste, touch and smell are functional. Touch, hearing, and memory tracks are laid down, learning, and memory develop. When you feel and live a healthy/happy life, memory is retained for a long time. Babies can learn in the womb and remember it well in later stages of life. This memory is called Implicit Memory.

The subconscious mind is dominant for the unborn baby and analysing the conscious mind is silent during pregnancy. By touching the mother's abdomen and talking, we can establish a strong bond with the unborn. Foetus learns language and emotions through the mother's voice. Heart sounds and bowel movement sounds are the nonstop background music in which the baby grows. That's why the baby strikes an immediate relationship with the mother on laying on the chest of the mother he hears the same background.

The Conscious Mind is called creative and it's the stage of self-learning like reading a book or going to a lecture, watching videos, or reading an article.

The subconscious mind is a habit mind. It's resistant to change, but we can reprogram the subconscious mind by erasing and self-destroying negative beliefs and reprogramming them with appropriate positive beliefs. With repeated affirmations and visualisations with strong intentions, the new belief gets strengthened and yields results.

So it's about habituation, erasing old beliefs and reprogramming with new beliefs is like weeding out negativeness.

Spiritual-Gold-Plating or Galvanoplasty

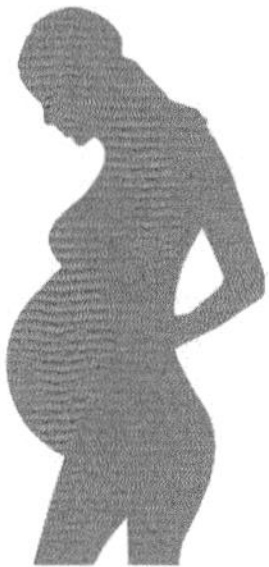

Mothers' thoughts pass through the bloodstream and reach the unborn in the womb, this is known as Spiritual-Gold-Plating or Galvanoplasty. If the mother has lofty thoughts and feelings - the baby will be healthy and beautiful.

The seed implanted in her womb may be of very exceptional quality, but if the mother has "leaden" thoughts in her head, she need not be surprised if later her child is cast in the lead that is vicious, pessimistic, or sick.

Once a child is born the dye has already been cast.

Music is the magical key that opens the heart and activates the brain, bringing tenderness and warmth into the heart and light and freedom into the mind.

Mohammed Ali, the world boxing champion says, "Champions are not made in the gym, it's made from desire, dream, and vision." His daughter Laila Ali Isa is a super middleweight champion. It's noted that offspring become pioneers in their father's fields. People say, it's in the blood, but it's more by nature of the family, genes, and the nurturing by the mother. The vision and desire of the mother, the unborn to be like her husband, and added grooming, play a major part in carrying the legacy of family sports like a relay game.

Touch the womb to boost his IQ, exercise to increase his IQ, and keep talking to the baby to get the best.

There are two types of Moms—
A mom who nurtures lovingly touching the unborn baby's head in the womb with strong bonding plus affirmations of love, care, and belief produces extraordinary and long-lasting results.

A managerial mom aims to have a genius child by commanding affirmations which are mechanical, bonding is weak, and belief only in achievement and skills.

Significance of a Father

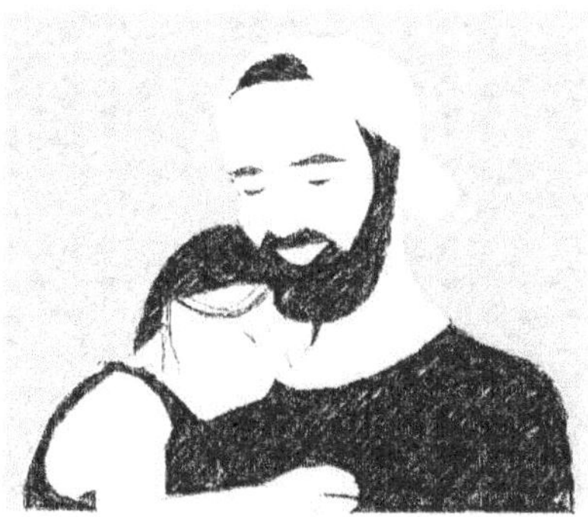

It's not flesh and blood alone, it's the heart that makes a father. The quality of a father can be seen in the goals he sets not only for himself but also for his family.

Loving touch to the womb, talking to the womb, soul seeding joy in you, create your future avatar Smarter and healthier unborn in the womb. In our culture, we designate it as Gharbhsamwad that's communicating with your womb.

True Story… Why?

It's only the child's potential that is reflected in their genes and not their fate.

The environmental variables influence 51% of a child's potential intellect, whereas genes account for 49% of the factors that determine IQ.

You must create certain conditions necessary for them to reach their full potential.

It should completely be the parents' to alter their perspective on life totally before welcoming a child.

According to research, when a mother is anxious, the baby's blood preferentially flows to the arms and legs, which results in smaller newborns and suppressed forebrain activity.

The development of children is facilitated by providing and caring for prenatal and perinatal surroundings as well as appropriate nutrition at a critical juncture in a child's development. The best growth booster is love, not the priciest school, the most expensive toy, or the highest-paying job.

On warm April and May days, parents were busy browsing for the best schools nearby. Looking for the best, looking for the affordable. Best schools are pricey, but they always have passionately committed teachers as they must get results from getting children on board as the students' results prove their efforts and good results attract parents to those institutions as they hope their children would become elite.

As the number of applicants increases, the institution toughens the norms of selection and monetizes the opportunity with all efforts.

In affordable institutions, teachers' passion to make their students the best and commitment are lacking because of a lack of support from the management. With all these discomforts some do become elite students.

With all the support, students are not elite, though, with poor institutional support, some do become elite....so, there is something more to be done...

Instead of running and spending on elite institutions, invest your time in the womb university, to get the best and desired progeny.

Progeny is the future generation. Every parent dreams of having desired progeny or genius, smart kids.

Is it possible? Do you want to have a genius, smart and healthy baby?

Testimonials can be narrated from mythology and the life of sports personalities as they reach the public limelight at an early age.

"Womb to Harvard" is a strategic vision to develop a vision for you to have your dream baby. The W2H uses the 1090 days strategy using various steps of motherhood.

Sparkle motherhood/ Womb motherhood/ Nutrition & protection motherhood/ Personality motherhood/ Achiever motherhood — it includes preconception to conception to birth to step to the soil to achieve.

Shall narrate to you a true story.

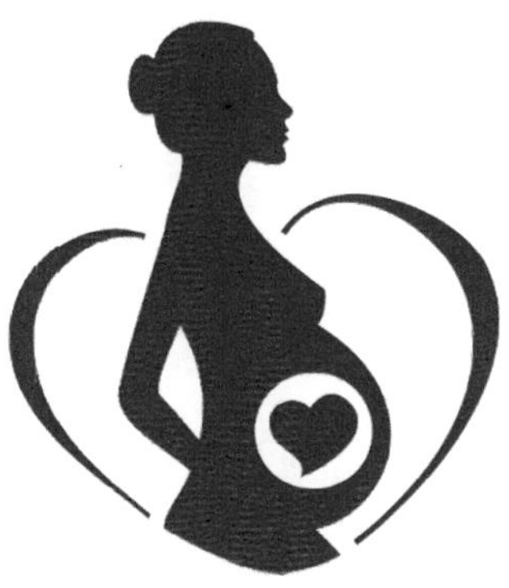

True Story

The Beginning of a Legacy
DR MANI PANCH

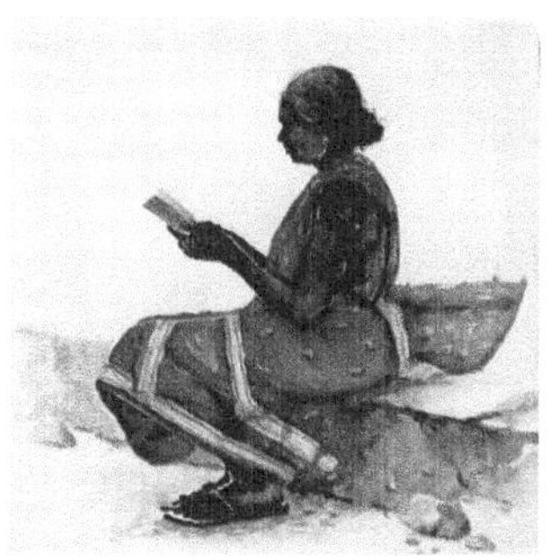

Shanthi was walking with a sundial (fried peas) in a basket around her waist and was visiting houses to disburse her orders for the day. Widower Shanthi with 3 children, 2 boys, and a daughter. Elder son Keshav was supporting his mother by working in a small shop, Mani, the younger son in school, and her baby daughter at home.

Mani was a good student, his dream was to become a Locomotive driver so he could travel all over the country.

Shanthi Amma was hoping her son Mani will get a decent salaried government job, he was going to a local school with hardships but was good in his studies.

She was discussing her family problems with her friend Parvathi and pinning her hope on her second son Mani.

Parvathi asked her what makes her confident that Mani will a helping hand.

"I got married at a very young age and had my elder son though I was quite ignorant my second pregnancy was a planned one wherein I had my grandmother to guide me throughout.

After conceiving, I was chanting Saraswathi Sthothram and reading Namam and was visiting temples frequently in the morning hours and had told him she needs him to study well and bring laurels to the family."

She told her friend she could feel his brilliance, her daughter

Paru was born when Mani was 2 years which was unplanned and Mani's father passed away suddenly.

Tears flowed and saw Mani coming from a school with long trousers, and a loose shirt stitched around the neck.

He was very loving to his mother, brother, and sister. He helps his mother, takes care of his sister, and is a responsible child.

His teachers appreciated his academic brilliance and everyone around him for his sense of society.

He used to stand near railway gates to see the Locomotives moving and dream of driving them one day.

He was good at playing football but he was more fond of reading books.

Wonders Happen…

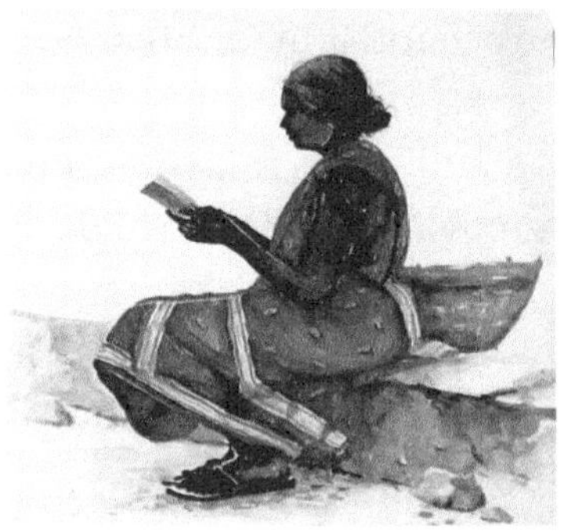

Mani completes his school with flying colors his mother asks him to go to Madras to get his Minimalist desire… to move the locomotive

He gets on a train and goes to Madras. His Mothers nurturing and affirmation brought unexpected fortunes

Mani joins college and his brilliance is reflected in classical singing, as he had a very commanding voice….

He started taking tuition for colleagues and classmates and all those who needed his coaching His communication and teaching skills were appreciated. He was using all these Skills for his living and to pay his fees for college, He was very generous and never indulged in any kind of dispute with anyone.

His academics as expected were brilliant. Nobody could believe that a boy from Socio Economically backwards society would be so academically well off and skillful at the same time. Many started appreciating him as a gem in the dust... some designated him as God's prodigy.

As the exams approached, he was cool as always when others were running for tuition, coaching... Mani was dreaming of his Locomotives....

He passed with flying colours in the final exam so his friend invited him to his home for a coffee to celebrate their success.

His friend Thomas had good results though not anywhere near Mani's. He accepted the invitation as he wants to meet his daddy to get guidance to go further to reach his goal to master locomotives.

He reached the big bungalow and stood in front of the gate and was hesitating to open the gate and enter as he had never gone to a bungalow or to any elite society gatherings.

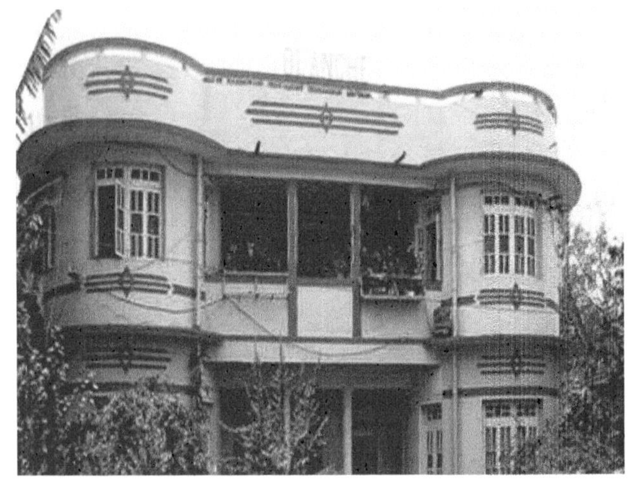

He started calling in low voice Thomas Thomas.... The front door opened and an aged person with spectacles visualised him and asked him "Yes son how can I help you?" Mani was surprised by his modesty and grandiose personality because his perception of elite people was to be proud and very commanding.

He replied, "Sir, I am Thomas's friend Mani," The man opened the full door to come and open the bungalow gate, he saw a man in a white coat over his shirt with a stethoscope in his side pocket. He came past his Land Master car parked on the porch of the house.

Mani for a second perplexed started imagining himself in this same outfit. He started loving the small Instrument hanging in his pocket...then he felt it was not for him. The poor boy has to limit his dreams and get back to the reality the doctor was Thomas's father.

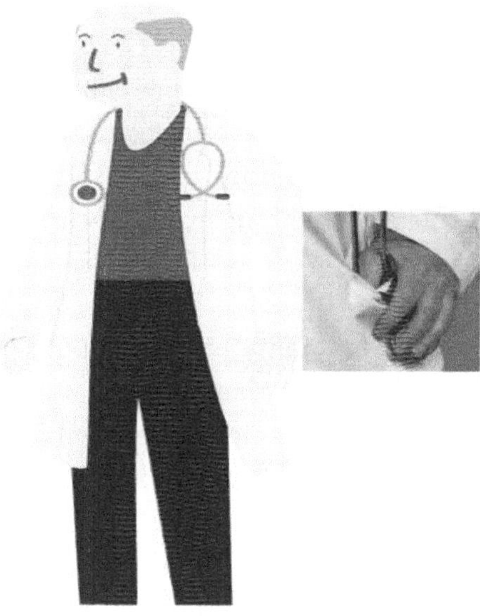

While greeting him in his drawing room, he saw the rich, beautiful drawing room, he sat on a very cosy sofa but was afraid his old pants could make the sofa dirty.

Thomas came dressed and introduced his father Dr. Bernard, Principal of Govt: Medical College, Madras.

In a casual discussion, Thomas told his daddy that Mani's intention is to Drive a Locomotive Engine and need advice for the same.

Then Dr. Bernard just casually enquired about his academic credentials!

Dr. Bernard's face facial expression was like an exclamation!!!! He moved a bit front in his seat and held Mani by his shoulder and patted Mani's face and said these credentials are to secure a seat at a Medical college.

Dr. Bernard told Mani that he should apply for Medical. He requested Mani to reconsider.
Mani was in tears and told Dr. Bernard Sir about his limits due to financial problems.

My old-aged mother and my elder brother with a petty job are supporting me and my baby sister after our father's demise. I have to support them as soon as I get a job.

Dr. Bernard was also moved mentally as he saw a hidden star or you can say a Diamond that needs polishing in front of him...

Bernard said, "Son, you can lose the opportunity. please understand."

Later, he enquired about his caste status though he knew they were socially backward and there was a government policy to support these communities.

In all aspects, be it credentials, community status, his admission to Medical College is more than 100% confirmed. He discussed with him everything in detail and said, "You qualify so much more than my son, and your ambition to support your mother, brother, and your baby sister and your community will be at a level which you cannot dream your status will be so high imagine Mani, you will be DRMANI PANCH... Add your father's credentials he will be a proud father wherever he is now... Your mother will feel so lucky to be a doctor's mother." Dr. Bernard motivated him.

Your vision is to explore India by driving the locomotive you will explore the world once you will receive all financial support from the government in the form of scholarships

I guarantee you and will support you throughout. Please discuss this with your mother and brother and be wise and bold to take the right decision.

I, Thomas and Sarkar are all with you maybe God sends me to you and I want his blessings to show you the right path. If it's meaningless so consider it as God's wish and put the responsibility on him and decide.

Mani was speechless hearing this wonderful angelic father-like God's Avatar in front of him. He touched Dr. Bernard's feet thanked me and said, "I will talk to my family and inform them of whatever you told me and by God's grace and by my mother's blessings, I will decide.

"Yes, I want to support my family in a better way and build a better social status for me and my community," he embraced. Thomas and I went to a coffee shop to celebrate.

In the coffee shop, he saw a man taking the juice out of the filter drawn out of coffee.

Coffee was squeezed into lot-a and tumbler with milk poured both of them pouring coffee

from the tumbler to lot-a, and vice versa mixing and cooling the coffee started sipping from the edge of the tumbler, Thomas encouraged Mani a lot And Mani decided to travel home to discuss with his Mother and elder brother.... He sat in a locomotive which was his dream... travelling to inform his mother of whatever Dr Bernard has told and he decided she and her brother take a decision.

Sound

gushed…IZIZIZIZ…CHUKCHUKCHUCHU…WITH SMOKE FROM THE ENGINE FROM

CHARCOAL BLACKENING AND FILLING THE SKY…Mani was moving to his hometown.

gushed…IZIZIZIZ…CHUKCHUKCHUCHU…WITH SMOKE FROM THE ENGINE FROM

Amma's Decision

Mani reaches the Victorian Architecture Railway station. From there he walked home and entered the lane leading from the town road to the community temple with a big banyan tree. He bowed to Ganesh under the banyan tree and bowed to the goddess and walked through the space between the banyan tree and temple to a community of more than 50 families staying in small walled houses.

Mani's home is a single-storeyed house with a sit-out veranda on the sides of the steps to the home where his family and community people gather with a tumbler of coffee and paper to discuss the events.

In town, ladies enquire about the release of new movies. As most ladies and children go together to movies mostly on Saturdays on Mondays with their husbands as it's a non-working day for the community.

It's a very vibrant community, they had common toilets, bathrooms, cloth washing area.

All these areas were gatherings of people discussing and enquiring about breakfast, a way to prepare, and movies, though sounds odd, the community communication was excellent and they stayed together…. for drinking water, they all had temple well. In the morning you could see ladies, children, and men helping each other with roping to fill the vessels for the day's water… they also fill the water tanks near the toilet, bathrooms, and cloth washing areas in turn for all their common use.

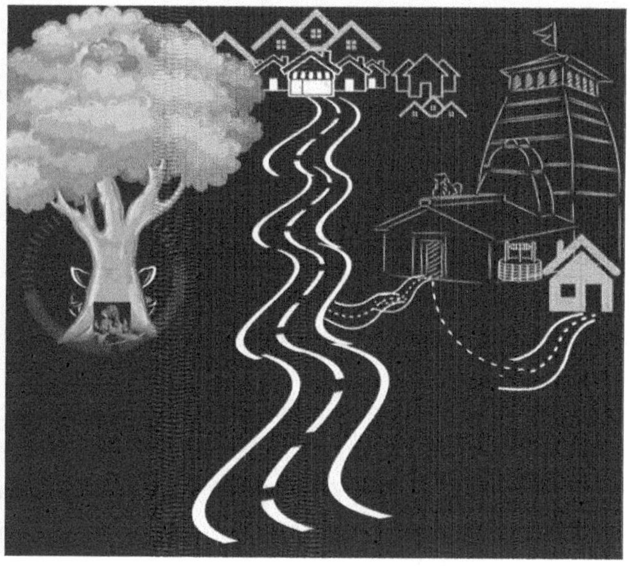

Everything in the community was temple centered. It was Devi Devi for the community they call her AATHA….MARIAMMA…

Mani saw his mother preparing the idly in a small wood-ignited kitchen pot and blowing it to increase the flame with water flowing from her eyes from smoke irritation. Mani came and hugged his Amma from behind without making any sound as she never knew of his coming. He said, "Amma…"

Shanthi turned and hugged her son. "Oh! Amma Mariyattha… I prayed to you, I wished my son was here and he is here and you made him appear here."

Mani was moved and he said, "You wish Amma, "*Devi*" will make me come here. I came to discuss important with you and anna but I will do it later. First, let me see my Anna and my sweet sis."

Anna Keshav hugged his thambi and said, "Mani you look weak; are you not eating properly?"

Mani smiles as Keshav always wants him healthier, and feels eating together with him, with ammas food only can keep him healthy. Mani told Keshav that he had an important discussion with his mother to decide on a very important matter regarding his studies. Mani said Anna whatever you and Amma will decide I'll follow it.

Baby sis Parvathi in a frock with a runny nose and cough came running to her chinna anna. Mani had her in his arms. He gave her sweets and *pedas* he had brought from Madras. He cleaned her up and put them on his lap Then all sat on the floor for the breakfast.

Shanthamma brought hot Idlis with coconut and chili chutney with sambar Everyone had it on their aluminum plate, laughing and chatting. Amma interrupted, "First eat and then talk."

"Shanthamma said most important thing is to see you all three together forever whatever the situation," she told Mani, "I want you to study well get a job earn a good income... take care of Keshav and Parvathi too."

Mani embraced and hugged his brother and sister and said, "Amma, anna and Paru are like you to me. Nothing in my life is more important than you," It was a lovely scene. Poverty doesn't affect the importance of living for each other.

As his anna was rushing to go shopping for work, Mani said, "Amma, I want to talk as anna, must be there for the discussion... anna will go and come back at night only before you would pack food for anna... Please amma come out of the kitchen for a while... it's very important."

Shanthamma was like *ennada periya vishayam* (what's the big matter), she giggled and said *ponnu ginny pathitya* (have any girl seen for you)

Mani said amma enough *Gelli amma* (no jokes ma).

Keshav came and held his mother by the hand and brought her out of the kitchen and all three sat in the small room on the floor as the house was with almost zero furniture. Though there was a wooden chair, Shanthamma always loved to sit with her children on the floor and chairs were kept for any guest who comes.

Mani started narrating all that happened in Thomas's house and Dr. Bernard's words, the government support and before he could finish and get to the discussion to decide Shanthamma and Keshav declared their decision in a single voice, hugged Mani and said, "Enga Mani Dr Mani Dhan...my Chinna paiyan (small boy) will be a doctor...Keshav my Chella thambi (loving brother) will be a doctor..."

Mani was perplexed and said amma it needs a lot of money to support me for the coming 5 years, how can we Amma?

Shanthamma and Keshav In a single voice said you will not only be the pride of the family but of our community. You can bring light and brightness to them and our temple. We both will work much more.

No second thought...Start your journey as a Doctor... Mani said amma let's talk about how we can afford or finance amma...Shanthamma and Keshav said you get ready to be a doctor

Paisa is our problem... Only Mariyattha...has come in the avatar of Dr Bernard, she has done her part... we will do ours, You finish your course and come... I never dreamt, you never dreamt Keshav never dreamt... but the goddess has dreamt... she will be with you... and we will accomplish our part...

Emotions, Pasam, Divine power... everything was flowing in harmony

Gods Epigenetics' embedding in Mani, He felt how blessed he was, and then he thought

Am I putting them into hardship...Keshav left to work. Before leaving he hugged you don't think of anything, I will manage... Enn Thambi Doctor Da9my brother doctor)... that chant in me will keep motivating me and amma... no more discussion you come back as a doctor and then we will talk...

MANI was in all sorts of emotions and prayed to god to be her son and his brother in another life or janam. He wrote a letter to Thomas and said he was coming and to follow his father's advice and informed him that his mother gives her vanakkam to his father and his mom sees Dr. Bernard as Devi's incarnation.

Mani was on his mother's lap ready to fly to the world of medicine. Shanthamma ran her fingers through Mani's curly hair… blessing and praying for the goddess to be with him every second and carry him in bright colours from all walks of life. "GODFATHER IN MAKING!"

Mani met all his neighbours and informed about his admission to medical college and promised them he will treat them all freely and be with them from all walks of life.

The Transformation

The White Coat-Medical Ragging-Bhagavathar

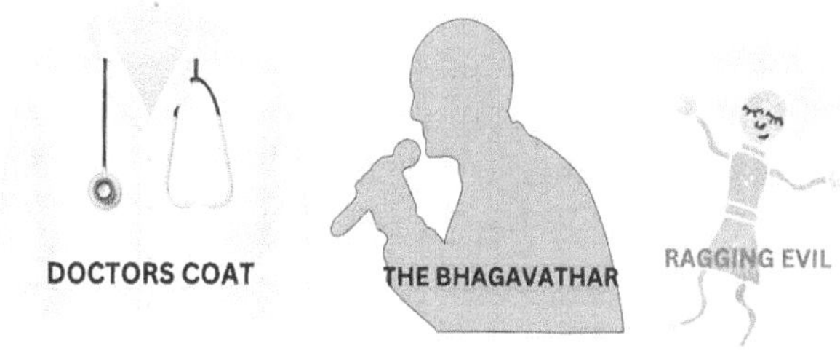

Mani dreams of chairing his mother in a golden chariot as the train moves, Mani thoughts of how his mother and brother will manage, his mind fighting "should I or should I not?"

But with his brother's words of his thambi doctor da and his mother's dream of seeing him as a community uplifter, he remembered the sparkle in her eyes, which indeed helped him to reach to a conclusion and end the battle of should I or should I not, at last, his inner voice said, "You must."

Wind flowing in the bogie and his thoughts coming out of conflict reassuring himself. He closed his eyes with the feeling of being in his mother's lap.

He walked into MMC (Madras Medical College), English touched victorian architecture, a noble college creator of millions of doctors and health workers.

Mani had two white coats and when he wore them the emotions and responsibilities, and values that the white coat holds, it felt overwhelming to him, just cannot be described in simple words.

A doctor's coat may seem ordinary and simple, but there is more to them than the eye. The white coat signifies cleanliness, knowledge, and authority. One requires all the traits in order to be a great doctor.

But unfortunately, Mani also had to undergo mental agony as a part of medical ragging.

In medical colleges, ragging refers to the practice of senior students putting newbies through a series of events and activities that are humiliating, embarrassing, and sometimes dangerous.

With a bit of careful planning, medical students can successfully navigate the challenges of ragging without succumbing to their negative effects.

But in Mani's case, ragging made them discover his talent for singing like a Bhagavathar.

He was not a trained classical singer. His mother said that she used to hear a lot of devotional songs like bhajans which are now exhibited in Mani. Now because of his bhajan singing, he was also known as Bhagavathar.

The raggers demanded him to sing *bhajans* that too in high-pitch trancing *bhajans*. Due to this, he had very little exposure to ragging.

As of now, the toughest phase in a medical career is the preclinical step. The three Frankenstein Foundations of Medical Science are human anatomy, human physiology, and human biochemistry.

Human anatomy was taught to illustrate the structure of human body organs.

Human physiology illustrates a functional aspect of the human body system.

Biochemistry to illustrate the chemical reactions involved in energy production, maintaining structural and functional integrity.

The three pillars of the medical foundation are as follows—

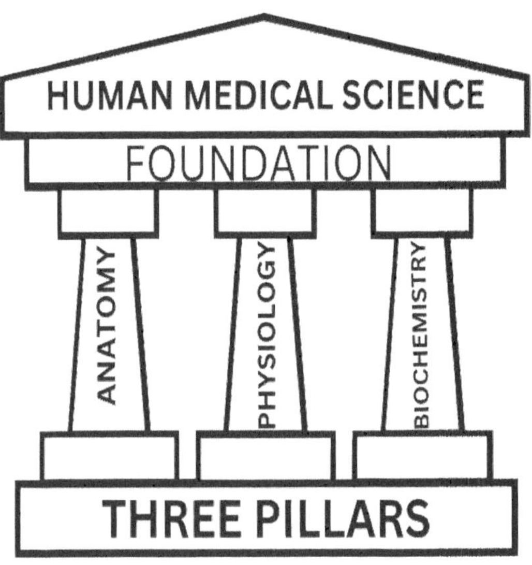

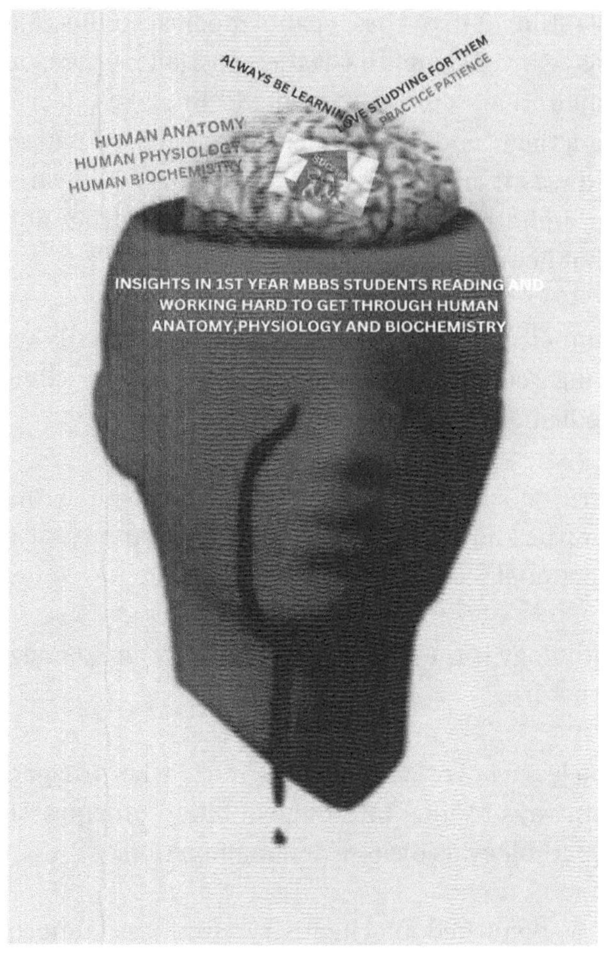

Insights: In 1st year, MBBS students read and work hard to get through human anatomy, physiology, and biochemistry.

As a student in the first year of medical studies, Mani was extremely enthusiastic, positive, brave, and explorative/ curious. He made mistakes, learned from them, and moved ahead. He practised patience and was thankful for what he got. He was aware of his limitations, but it did not stop him from doing what he wanted to.

Mani crossed the barrier of 1st year of MBBS with flying colours entering the world of clinical medicine to 2nd year of medicine.

Here you interact with humans and you witness how the knowledge is used to identify structural and functional pathology.

Pathology is the disturbed physiology and damaged structure.

You learn how senior doctors and teachers diagnose pathways to illustrate the exhibition of expression of pathology as disease and malfunction.

How disturbed biochemistry produces abnormal elements which are used as markers of pathology or disease pharmacy you learn.

To use medicines and how they are used to treat and their adverse effects. As the years passed by Mani was marveling at the truth of modern medicine.

Mani's amma, anna, sis Paru, and the whole community were looking up to Mani to bring laurels to the community and family.

45

Happy Events & Dr. Thambi

Mani was immersively working in the wards as he entered his pre-final year training. Warden had sent the peon enquiring for Mani as he had letters from home. It was a letter from *amma* requesting him to come home for two days as his presence was of utmost importance.

He sprinted to the college office and applied for two days' leave. This is the first time Mani was taking off during his working hours. It was granted and he rushed to Madras Central Railway Station. On the way, he purchased flowers and sweets for his sister, mom & brother. He got into the general compartment with much difficulty as it was the Christmas holiday season.

He arrived home the next morning, everyone now designates him as Doctor Thambi before everyone calls him Mani Thambi. Now Mani felt something in him and he can see the smile on Shanthammas' face, a cheerful face of completeness or achievement.

Mani wondered why so many people gathered in front of his house. Shanthamma told him his sister has become a mature girl.

Mani ran to see his sister, his kutty sis with shyness and in thavani attire, he couldn't control his tears of happiness, seeing his sister as a woman.

He just prodded his hands on his sister, blessed her, and got her head closer and lay on his shoulder and chest as if promising her, 'I am there'. Shanthamma and Kesav joined the hug and all of them felt Mani's warmth and care. Paru fell on Mani's feet for his blessings and Kesav pulled her and looked at Shanthamma and resonated, "Amma, Paru..did you hear it's not only me the whole community designates him as Doctor Thambi? I am so proud of Mani to be your brother."

Mani places a hand on Kesav's mouth and says, "It's the other way anna. I am blessed with such a loving brother," and touches his anna's feet for blessings.

It was a moment of pride for Shanthamma when everyone designated her son as Doctor Thambi, the function went on, as this function informs the community of a girl maturing into a woman and will mature to get married and all families will consider the girl when they think of their son's marriage.

Every woman in the community participates and in queue puts tilak on Paru's forehead and everyone brings sweets and small gifts. The entire family has food together and departs blessings to Paru.

Mani said, "Amma, get Kesav anna a good girl to get married."

Shanthamma said, "I am already looking for him."

Mani said, "Amma, in one year, I will complete my medical school education, then I will be on horsemanship for a year during which he will get stipend money, then he will come back to be with her forever." Shanthamma said "Mani, study more Mani said no amma I have to come back to take care of you all and back to my community to serve them as well. Don't worry amma; you, anna, and our community goddess Panchariaiamman have blessed me with something I never dreamt of. Now it's my turn to keep you all happy and our goddess' poojas and celebrations go on well."

Shanthamma held Mani closer, kissed his forehead and told him "Mani, you will be not only Doctor Thambi, but you are also born to be a Thaliavar... yes the legend was on making."

Till now it was all the making of Doctor Thambi; the beginning of the legacy starts but before I go forward, we have to analyze the tools that happened in the shaping of Doctor Thambi. Here we need not look into other families, in the same family three children with the same genes but expressions were different.

The fact that we are a continuation of the DNA and impressions left on us by our parents and ancestors. The continuity of human existence may be found in the body on a physical level and in the mind on a programme level.

The programme is referring to the innate characteristics of the person's personality. The mother's diet, thoughts, speech, and actions affect the fetus. child combines three phenomena its own destiny/parental traits/pregnancy care.

Analysis & Conclusion

The above story is a true story of a legend though the legend is no more he made an ecosystem of a family of doctors, through his sons, sons-in-law, grandsons & daughters, highly qualified & salaried computer stalwarts working independently in the USA, in Apple & Google, granddaughter with Ph.D. & her husband and IAS both now studying at Harvard, the legend Dr. Mani lives in every one of them.

Manis' last journey in his home town even nature poured the tears as rain. He grew from the unknown to the best known and created an ecosystem in his family with a highly educated, skilled generation.

It all started in the Shanthamma womb. It all started with preconception planning, womb caring, talking, postnatal care, and seeding the right thoughts and culture to the children's minds and the environment were the epigenetic Factors that changed the expression of ordinary Mani to the Dr. Thambi to Dr. Thalaivar to doctor the godfathers. The legend was made.

I will analyse and explain the tools that caused epigenetics of the above portion of the story and then take you to the next part of the story "Doctor Thalaivar" & then to the third part "Doctor Thatha the godfather".

Let's move to tools to understand how we can change genetic expression to achieve our desired progeny.

To know More about the Section, Scan the Code

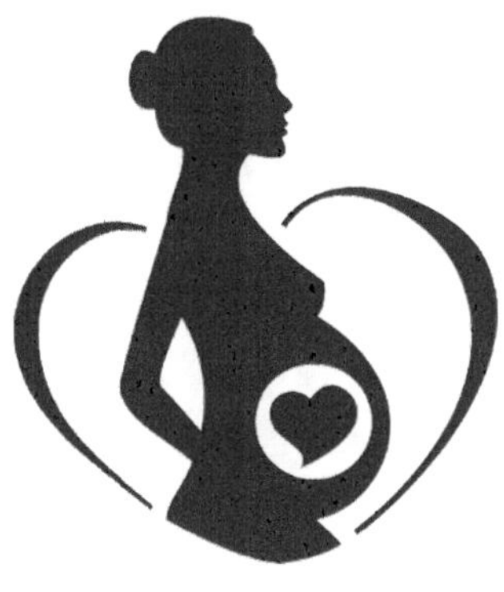

Section 2

The first classroom is the womb, and the second classroom is the environment you provide after the child is born. So when the child attends pre-school, it would have been to two schools before pre-school. The journey of learning starts before we are born.

Preface

"The Womb to Harvard "

From conception till 3 years of age. Give your child the best chance at success with a customised plan for their life. Learn more about personalised development plan and how it works. Help your little one reach their full potential with womb to Harvard university.

Experience-based

Babies hear familiar voices and music in the womb and are comforted by them after birth. The rocking motion of vehicles may remind unborn babies of their mother's body, soothing them.

Repetition

If a mother repeats conversations with the child in utero, it may respond immediately.

Associative learning

The baby may associate what you say with how you feel. If you're sad and talking to your baby in the womb, those words are also sad. Similar patterns apply to other emotions.

The mother/daily caregiver's conversations and experiences affect the fetus development. Direct foetus prenatal engagement may improve mental health and pregnancy's self-efficacy. To conclude, the baby in the uterus is hearing all the noises from the environment, the hidden and subconscious learning may be impacting their growth and development. In a peaceful surrounding, prenatal baby talk as learning is innate and has no age or boundary for its inception start the prenatal baby talk.

From conception to 3 years of age.

Give your child the best chance at success with a customized plan for their life.

Learn more about our personalised development plan and how it works.

Help your little one reach their full potential from Womb to Harvard University.

Let me start with what made me write this book.

The Story.
She opened my mind to write this book. The author narrates—

"'Aya Pakkanum Aya pakkanum' in Tamil "I want to see, Sir," it was a lady talking to my wife.

I came out and saw she was our colony cloth ironing lady's daughter.

I remember seeing her 18 years or so on her baby shower day. I went to her and saw her in tears as she talked to my wife. The moment she saw me her voice grew thinner and tears flowed and her eyes and facial expression proved its tears of joy, she reacted "Doctor Aya! Being a Paediatrician and Neonatologist, I enquired about anything wrong with the kids. She shook no and was almost to my feet, I held her.

I remember on the day of her baby shower when she came to take blessings from me and my wife she said, "Dr Aya bless me to have a son who will be a doctor like you."

I smiled and told her, "Son or daughter, your baby will become a doctor, pray to god, talk to your womb baby and make him know your desire, and you visualise him to be a doctor and he gets your vision." I said belief in yourself and I went back to KSA, where I was working at that time.

Time passed, pages of life turned, and now I am a grandfather of four grandchildren.

I used to see her son helping his mom and at times I see him sitting under the ironing trolley and reading. As my car passed before their trolley on my way back from the hospital I inquired if he was fine.

She said, "Ayah, your blessings have come true, my son has completed his NEET and is now selected for AIIMS, DELHI," I asked her, "What me?"

She said, "You blessed and advised me. I prayed to God and kept on talking to him whenever I saw doctors. I visualised and told him how he will look in that attire now he will wear it." I was stuck not knowing how to react, as it was a casual blessing and parental tip.

I told her "God is great and you are a Mother Achiever, and his son is so lucky to have a mother like you."

She said, "Ilaya (no sir), it was your advice and I felt even financially and people like us can dream by nurturing our hopes in the womb and my prayers with trust in him and belief in myself I can do it."

It was a moment of joy and that lady opened my eyes, I know about them and their background, very few of them even pass out of school. Her nurturing, talking, and visualising had worked wonders.

Epigenetics is the science of how the environment influences the rearrangement of DNA Genes."

In stages of the embryo, the mind is deeply attached to its parents. Whatever she listens to with attention contributes to culturing the mind of the child

We call PARENTS AS "GENETIC ARCHITECT"

In the book and course "Womb to Harvard University" the author's mission is to create millions of parental architects and groom them from the womb stage, even before.

"WOMB TO HARVARD UNIVERSITY"

The signature name of the book can be "Womb to Oxford", "Womb to Princeton", "Womb to Royal College", "Womb to AIIMS", and so on.

Destinations can be any or different, but the starting point is only one, "the womb or the womb university".

"One good mother is worth a hundred schoolmasters."

—George Herbert.

Womb Harmonics, Nurturing and Caring for those nine months of the womb, with additional rituals will create virtues in the unborn baby from THE WOMB TO BIRTH A GENIUS "WITH HIGHER IQ, EQ, SQ AND AQ*

In this section, we will be empowering knowledge of progeny, epigenetics, advantages of the unborn, water media, preconception guidelines, different stages of motherhood, effects of nutrition, exercises, and sound and methods of nurturing all in a simple and practical mode and much more.

**"The smile that flickers on a baby's lips when he sleeps- does anyone know where it was born?
Yes, there is a rumour that a young pale beam of a crescent moon touched the edge of a vanishing autumn cloud, and there the smile was first born in the dream of a dew-washed morning."**

—Rabindranath Tagore

Epigenetics

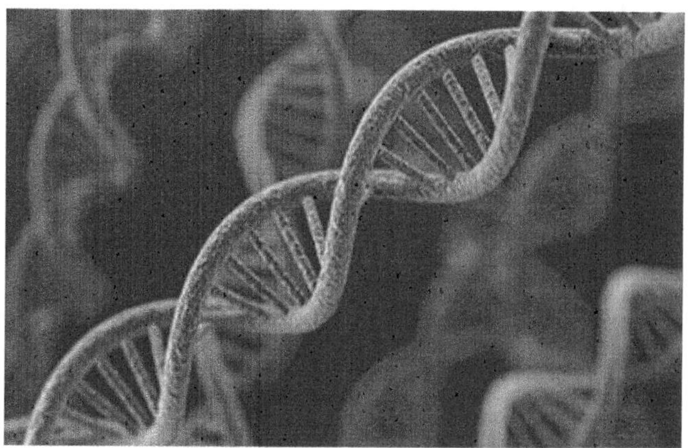

It's a science or process of gene expression modified without affecting the basic gene structure. Simple and best way to understand. Wild forest elephants or tigers. Gene expression is wild, but by providing a different environment training and different socialising methods their gene expression changed to a domestic obedient animal. Though like the wild animal, the tamed animal genes are the same. The expression of the gene influenced by the environment changed their expression. This process or science of changing gene expression is the science of epigenetics.

"Change in phenotype without a change in genotype."

DNA isn't your destiny, it's your expression.

What Is Epigenetics?

"The new science of epigenetics reveals how the choices you make can change your genes and of your kids." Foods we eat, our sleeping patterns, and chemicals in the environment, can impact gene expression. Cells are fundamental working units of every human being. All the instructions required to direct their activities are contained within DNA. Genes are specific sequences of bases that provide instructions on how to make important proteins.

DNA from humans is made up of approximately 3 billion nucleotide bases. Within the 3 billion bases, there are about 20,000+ genes.

Genes are specific sequences of bases that provide instructions on how to make important proteins. A "genome" is an organism's complete DNA set, including all its genes. Each genome contains all the information needed to build and maintain that organism

Role Of Epigenetic In Unborn Baby

A large amount of scientific evidence indicates that life experience can affect gene expression — how information in a gene is used (epigenetics) — in some cases by slowing or shutting the genes off, and in others by increasing their output. This is why identical twins are not carbon copies of each other. Although their genes (DNA code) are identical, their epigenetic markers are different from birth and continue to diverge as they interact with the environment in distinctive ways. Even more important, these epigenetic changes can be permanent and passed down from generation to generation.

In the age-old nature-versus-nurture debate, epigenetics offers a surprising middle ground.

A baby in the womb is not just a clump of cells. It is also the tiny human being that is growing inside you. During pregnancy, your baby is influenced by many factors to ensure he or she becomes a healthy child. We explore some of the ways an unborn baby is influenced by his or her mother during pregnancy and what this means for his or her future health as an adult.

Prenatal Diet

Pregnancy diets can affect epigenetics. Epigenetic factors are food nutrients. These nutrients help your baby grow. Epigenetic factors include: Pregnancy food can also affect your unborn child. The baby needs iron and folic acid.

These nutrients affect fetal epigenetics:

Vitamin B9: aids brain development in babies. It enhances elderly cognitive function.

Vitamin B12: Your baby needs this vitamin for red blood cell and brain DNA synthesis. Folate: Your baby's nervous system and brain need folate. Iron: Your baby's brain and DNA need iron.

Zinc: Your baby's nervous system and brain need zinc.

Pregnancy Exercise
Pregnancy benefits from exercise.
Regular exercise during pregnancy reduces the risk of maternal complications like high blood pressure, gestational diabetes, preeclampsia, and Cesarean section, according to numerous studies. Regular exercise prevents obesity and maternal depression.

Pregnancy Hormone Prolactin
It aids lactation and baby development.

Thyroid Hormones:

They help your unborn baby's brain and metabolism develop. Pregnancy raises thyroid hormone levels.

Oestrogen:

Pregnancy's main female sex hormone.

It develops your uterus, placenta, and blood vessels. They aid baby development. Pregnancy hormone oxytocin. It aids baby development. Pregnancy produces the stress hormone cortisol. It helps your baby grow

Conclusion:

During pregnancy, your baby is exposed to many substances that can affect the epigenetics in his or her genes. Certain nutrients found in foods are called epigenetic factors.

These nutrients are important for your baby's development.

Progeny

(Generations Inheritance)

Genealogy refers to the offspring of a couple. An individual's progeny are those people who share their genetic makeup. Our children and grandchildren are the "PRIDE OF THE FAMILY & SOCIETY." Nonetheless, these days we discuss genetics and DNA...

Before or when genetics was not understood

They understood that a strong, attractive offspring relied on a strong, attractive parent. So strong men married beautiful women and vice versa. The result was a stunningly attractive and formidable new generation, but at the cost of a weaker, lower-profile human society and the emergence of new divisions among civilisations.

The dominant culture convinced the submissive culture that it would sacrifice everything for the weaker culture, and the submissive culture obliged. They rose to power, and those in positions of authority avoided having children with members of less dominant societies for fear of diluting their power. So royals married royals, and the practice became institutionalised as a legacy by the fact that Royals, Parivar, Tharavads, made it forbidden to form partnerships with members of lower social classes. The members of the Power Society were aware that they could not rely only on their power or the beauty or physical power of females and males respectively to get the best, hence they experimented with a variety of methods to bring out the best in themselves.

Men's abilities were put to the test, much like India's Swayamvar, to help them marry a beautiful woman. They also resorted to astrology, numerology, and spirituality to help them have best progeny. From what we can tell, the ultimate goal of all cosmic creation was to produce healthy, intelligent, and smart offspring. The potential IQ of your offspring is not fixed by any one factor.

The Key

Teaching the fetus that you want it to be a master, teach it repeatedly. If a book is read aloud repeatedly if recorded, play it repeatedly for a time and move to the next level. Do it with passion and appreciation. That's the key.

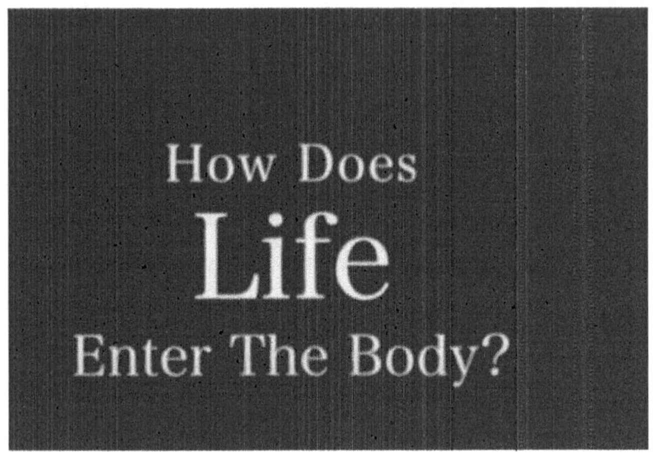

Theory Of Life In Force

This life force is free and independent and enters the embryo of its own will. Thus, the creation of a new life is considered to be no less than a natural miracle!

When sperm meets the ovum, the result doesn't need to become an embryo. Conception only occurs when the life force also enters the seed and fuses with them at the same time, giving rise to the live embryo. We must understand and realise this. Right after this rush of life force, comes the formation of the baby's mind.

Spirit or soul entering an unborn baby during conception is the process by which a spiritual entity enters an unborn child and remains with it for the remainder of its life. It is a common belief in many cultures that a person's spirit or soul will enter their new-born child if they are pregnant with them, and this is a practice known as *prenatal spirit communication*. This could be something good for you ,your prayer to God may have been answered. The spirit usually enters into the fetus at about 30 days of pregnancy; however, it can happen earlier than that, and it can also happen after the fetus has been born. If the spirit stays, it will stay with you until you leave this world.

- There are many theories surrounding the topic of whether a human being can have both a physical body and a soul. *Researchers, doctors, and philosophers have spent years investigating this concept. Several experts and organizations recognize that not everyone accepts scientific evidence on the subject of life and consciousness.* However, there is *widespread acknowledgment that science cannot yet explain everything about how our minds function or why we have emotions, thoughts or a sense of self.* There are many myths surrounding life after death. *The belief that our souls live on after we die is called spiritism, spiritualism, or paranormal activity.* Understanding what happens when a person dies and the soul entrer into an unborn baby during conception is important for everyone who believes in an afterlife.

- There are various beliefs about the nature of human spirits. Some believe that a human being has a soul and is made up of a spirit, while others believe that a human being has a spirit and is made up of a soul. Presently, we observe at both sides of the argument to understand if the spirit or soul enters the unborn baby during conception

Water and Spirituality

The unborn interacts with the mother by reverberation property of amniotic fluid, when the foetus is submerged in water for 270 days in the womb. The mother nurtures her unborn child by speaking to, stroking, and feeling her unborn child.

In a single sentence, what is reverberation?

The persistence of sound after a sound is made is referred to as reverberation in acoustics. Due to the presence of numerous reflecting surfaces, a single sound experiences numerous reflections.

Organs like the brain contain roughly 80% water, while the average human body is about 70% water. Every cell in our body is made up of water. Hindus, Christians, and Muslims, respectively, believe in the divinity and spirituality of water, which makes up 72% of our body structure and is essential to the smooth operation of every system. Other places where this belief is shared include the Ganges and Teerth, the Grotto of Massabielle in the sanctuary of Our Lady of Lourdes, and ZamZam water from Mecca. We think that by consuming these spiritual and holy fluids, our bodies will be rejuvenated and purified.

Water has the important property of REVERBERATION.

The characteristics and uses of water in the natural world are better-understood, (*thanks to science!*).

How we preserve, safeguard, and distribute the water resources of Earth are decisions *influenced by ethics.*

SPIRITUALITY aids us in determining our fundamental beliefs regarding the significance and worth of water

Water, a component of the natural world, has long served as the focal point of spiritual symbolism and religious ceremony in human civilizations.

Water has been employed by human societies to convey the sacredness of life, the spiritual significance of purification, protection, and healing, as well as the profound significance of suffering and atonement in human life.

Water in Ritual and Symbol
Hindus in India view the Ganges as a manifestation of the goddess Ganga. This makes the Ganges River

a representation of life as well as a location where one can purify their soul and go closer to the divine source of life. One drop of water is provided by the Science of Teerth temples, which even a multi-millionaire covets because it is unavailable elsewhere. Water is what reminds us of the divine. Teerth is exactly this. To be reminded of their divinity, people desire to consume it.

An ancient Jewish custom commands people to immerse in a "mikvah" bath to spiritually cleanse their bodies on certain occasions. In Roman Catholicism, for instance, water can be ritually sanctified and used as a symbolic representation of God's protection over anybody or everything touched by the Holy Water. Catholics frequently make the Sign of the Cross when they enter (for cleansing) and depart (for protection) a church by dipping the fingers of their right hand into a Holy Water fountain. When doing their morning prayers, many Eastern Orthodox Christians either sip a tiny bit of blessed water or sprinkle a little holy water over their food as they cook.

For Muslims, wudu, or ablution with water, is a required pre-prayer ritual. In the Qur'an, the prophet Mohammed says: "O you who believe! When you stand up for prayer, wash your cheeks, wipe your head, and wash your hands up to your elbows (5:6). Islam uses water as a metaphor for the various stages of life. Most importantly, believers will arrive in a garden of paradise with cold streams and springs of fresh drinking water at the end of the journey. According to the Qur'an, believers would benefit from "rivers of non-stagnant water" and "a flowing fountain" (47:15). (88:11-12).

Water is memory, it makes up 72% of your body, which is what makes you physically exist. As a tall bottle, we are. Making a vessel's water nice will also make our water more pleasant.

Why is water important in Womb to Harvard Strategy?

Unborn lies in the womb in water based medium, completely immersed, and with the *reverberant property of water.* It's easy to nurture the baby by sound and touch to teach him, get connected to him, express your desires and nurture and mould him to be what you desire.

Motherhood

Marriage

Motherhood is healthier after marriage. Marriage is a culturally significant and frequently legally recognised relationship between two people who are referred to as spouses. It is also known as matrimony and wedlock.

It sets forth the rights and responsibilities that each party owes to the other, as well as to their children and their in-laws.

In Hinduism, a religious marriage is referred to as *vivah* or *kalyanam*, in Catholicism, is referred to as a sacramental marriage; in Islam, it is called *nikah*; in Judaism, it is called *nissuin*; and various other names are used for religious marriages in other faith traditions. Each of these religions has its own set of rules regarding what constitutes a valid religious marriage and who is eligible to enter into one.

The condition of being married and even the act of tying the knot are all considered valid definitions of the term "matrimony." The root 'matri' is derived from the Latin word 'mater', for "mother"; the suffix

- money refers to a state of being, a function, or a role.

Therefore, entering into a marriage is the state that transforms a woman into a mother demonstrating the degree to which the processes of reproduction and child-rearing are fundamental to the institution of marriage.

In Canon 1055 of the code of Canon Law, it is stated that "the matrimonial covenant, by which a man and a woman establish between themselves a partnership for the whole of life, is by its nature ordered toward the good of the spouses and the procreation and education of offspring."

The voluntary willingness of a man and a woman to enter into marriage is typically referred to as "matrimonial consent," and the term is frequently used in this context. This highlights the legal, contractual, or covenant aspect of marriage, which is why, in addition to being used to signify the sacrament of marriage, the term "matrimony" is still widely used today in legal references to marriage. This emphasises the degree to which reproduction and socialisation are intertwined with marriage.

Sparkle Mother: Lights the Next-Gen in Her Womb
It's the preconception process that creates a sparkle mother who conceives the light of the future.

3 months before conception in order to ensure the fetus has the best possible chance of reaching its full potential, but others may use the term "women's health" interchangeably.

Even before they become pregnant, parents-to-be should start devoting time and energy to planning for their child so that they can increase the likelihood that they will have a child who is healthy, intelligent, and well-versed in their culture. The one and only solution that aims to ensure that future generations will be intellectually more advanced and possess a greater variety of characteristics. Cells that are not only healthy but also capable of reproduction give attention to the young seedlings, putting the pieces of the environment together.

All of the following should be present in order for conception to take place: sperm that is well-formed and of high-quality sperm, a healthy ovum, a healthy and robust uterus, a fertile period in the woman's cycle, and a cultured soul that is full of good deeds. In order for the woman to have a successful pregnancy, it is imperative that she ensures that she is getting the proper amount of nutrition. Before starting a family, both men and women should strive to realise their full potential in terms of their physical and mental well-being. This is a prerequisite for family formation. Having a higher risk of being frail, having fewer attractive features, and living for a shorter amount of time is associated with having children that were conceived with poor-quality sperm.

Before trying to conceive a child, it is important for both the man and the woman to maintain a healthy lifestyle and diet. Consuming foods such as dates, raisins, pomegranate, soaked figs, leafy vegetables like spinach, and other foods rich in similar nutrients is especially important for women who wish to raise their haemoglobin levels and nourish their blood.

It is recommended that women listen to particular genres of therapeutic music in order to achieve mental and physical equilibrium.

It is important to avoid negative emotions such as grief and irritation as well as depression, disappointment, and stress because these might have a negative impact on the quality and quantity of both sperm and eggs. This is why it is important to steer clear of negative emotions.

When sperm and an egg come into contact with one another, there is no assurance that an embryo will develop as a result of this interaction. The process of conception cannot begin until the life force also reaches the seed and combines with it at the same time. As a direct consequence of this, a living embryo will be formed.

When fertilisation takes place, also known as the process that forms the embryo, there is already a distinct mind present in the developing embryo.

Womb Mother-300 Golden Days-Gods Own Secret

Human development begins at conception, when a woman and man unite 23 of their own chromosomes. At conception, sperm and egg combine to form a single-cell embryo. This embryo holds a new person's genetic information. Fertilization determines gender, eye colour, and other features. In the first eight weeks after conception, most body parts and systems exist and begin to operate. The head, chest, abdomen, pelvis, arms, and legs form four weeks after conception. Except for size, the developing human's look and internal structures resemble a new-born at 8 weeks.

Pregnancy isn't simply about body growth. It's also a moment for post-birth survival. Frequent everyday activities start in the womb more than 30 weeks before birth. Hiccups, stroking the face, breathing motions, urine, right or left-handedness, thumb-sucking, swallowing, yawning, jaw movement, reflexes, REM sleep, hearing, taste, feeling, etc.

A full-term pregnancy lasts 38 weeks from conception or 40 weeks from the woman's last period.

Learning Inside The Womb

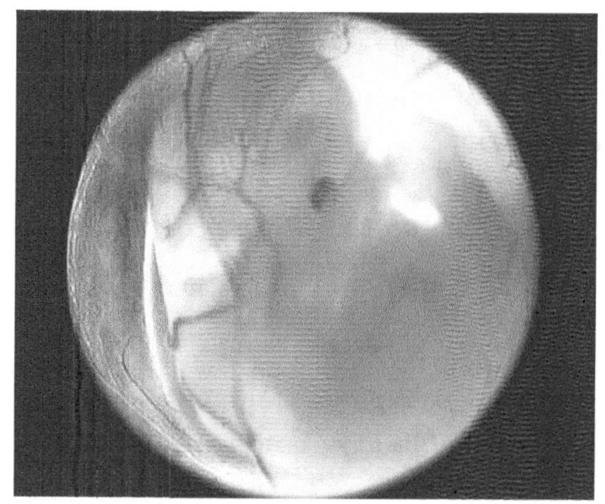

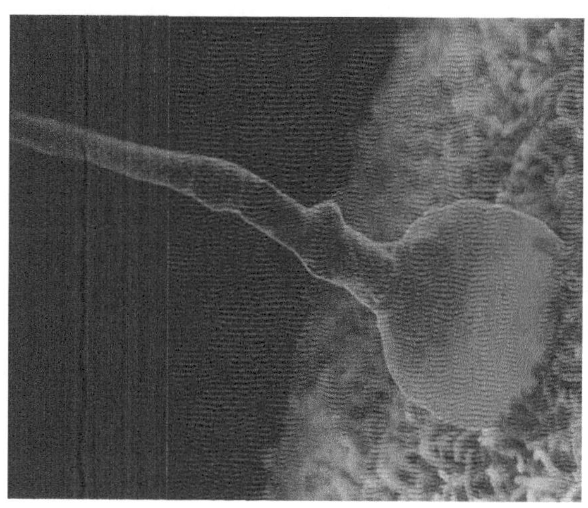

In this section, your unborn says about his development and explains the events occurring in Mother's womb.

Let's see the womb from that fetus'perspective.

1. (1st Trimester)

Every ounce of genetic information, from hair colour to piano talent, resides in a single cell after 24 hours. Again, we divide. After a week in the ovaries, *we split in two in the uterus*. The *other half forms the placenta, which provides food, oxygen, and waste removal.*

By the 4th week, we're a 1 million-cell-per-second-growing tiny being. Even as a *poppy seed*, our spinal cord, heart, and brain are evident.

2. (1st Trimester)

We're 10,000 times bigger than at conception when the heartbeat begins.

This is crucial in our neurological development, as the brain generates 100,000 cells every minute. Our brain can be affected by the consumption of our mother's alcohol or drugs, and inducing stress or trauma. This can cause math issues or schizophrenia 40 years later.

If mom stays healthy and relaxes, our brain can grow *raspberry-sized.*

3. (1st Trimester)

We start reacting to stimuli around month 3.

Our sense of smell is developing and pollutants can be unpleasant. Our brain grows quickly. Soon, we can hear our mom's heartbeat and voice. Still small, the tummy has lots of room. Our *sensory playground is the womb.* We stretch our arms, smile, and thumb-suck. 75% prefer the right hand. We're *lemon-sized.*

4. (2nd *Trimester*)

Half of our size is head. Kicking, peeing, and swallowing are taught. Developing taste buds. *If our mother eats a variety of foods, we become less picky eaters.*

If we have insufficient nutrition, our bodies adjust to continue growing. This is foetal programming. This can lead to obesity, heart disease, and diabetes later in life, say researchers. We're as large as a *tomato.*

5. (2nd Trimester)

Our *mom's muffled voice is becoming clearer.* We experience a growth spurt and start developing teeth, hair, fingernails, eyebrows, and eyelashes. We're become more active and love exercising our muscles. *As we move, our mother will feel us. If she answers, we learn every action has a reply.* We're now *dragon fruit-sized.*

6. (2nd Trimester)
The cerebral cortex separates into two hemispheres in the sixth month.

But it's also exciting because our eyes open. We respond to light despite seeing merely blurs. *Some suggest our mom should take us outside now.* We're making simple facial gestures like a "grin." When we're born and desire to display our feelings, we probably learn to communicate. We're like a little *cauliflower.*

7. (3rd Trimester)
We develop regular sleep-wake cycles. Our hair is now apparent and milk teeth have emerged. *When we hear our mom, our heartbeat and movement may rise. Some studies say we learn language from outside sounds. We prefer our parents' native language once born.* Having a 90% chance of surviving if born now, *Pineapple-sized.*

8. (3rd Trimester)
We've become infantile. The brain and nerve system are ready. We're practising breathing by inhaling amniotic fluid. We spend practically all our time sleeping and thinking about the future. Most have

turned upside down in preparation for birth. Our bones and skull are flexible to fit through the tunnel's tiny aperture. The immune system is young. Our internal bodyguards won't be fully effective for months following birth.

Now we're *melon-sized.*

9. (3rd Trimester)

We've been training motor skills and kicks this month. When our mom laughs, consume sweets or drinks ice tea, we may bounce. If we could interpret study articles, we'd hope for a normal birth to give us a stronger immune system for life. The riddle of nature vs nurture is well-begun and reveals our character. Early childhood is the missing piece.

We're *jackfruit-sized* after 9 months.

As the unborn had explained his journey in the womb, the mother has to perform month-wise to support the unborn as this is the best time to make him healthy, brainy, smart and loving. So follow the monthly wise activities to get your desired baby.

Your unborn baby will be what you desire, pray to God talk to your womb baby and make him know your desire, and you visualise him to be as desired and he gets your vision... believe in yourself

Every nutrition is for his specific monthly growth, listening to music, practising skills every day like drawing, weaving sweaters for baby, doing creative activities, visualising how your baby to be, keep him as a friend and talk to him, tell him stories good ones, push in your desires into him with love which stimulates the organo-genesis and his subconscious mind accepts and he responds with movements. I will explain on a monthly basis, and follow as much as possible.

Month 1 (1st Trimester)

In 24 hours of Life

Nutrition.
Gooseberry. Lime. Lemon. Pomegranate. Orange. Sweet lime. Black gram. Seasonal produce.

- Fluids. Water Or milk?
- Green gram water drained.
- Soup.
- Clothes.
- White and pastel-colored slacks.
- Ornament
- Diamond, silver.
- Reading.
- Spiritual reading and praying
- Entertainment.
- 20-minute garden walk.
- Soft music.
- Worship.
- Contraindication.
- Spicy fried food.
- Beverages. Dry, stale food. Non-edible.
- Traveling.
- Weightlifting.
- 8-week development
- Half-inch baby.

- The nose tip and eyelids are forming.
- Well-formed arms and legs.
- Longer, clearer fingers and toes.

2. (1st Trimester)

If the mom drinks, uses drugs or endures tremendous stress or trauma, the baby's brain can be affected. It can cause math issues or schizophrenia 40 years later. If the mom stays healthy and relaxes, the baby's brain can grow.

Nutrition.

- Moderately. Spicing.
- Liquid-based food.
- Lotus stem water.
- Chestnut. Watermelon. Rice, semolina, beaten rice, and broken wheat porridge.
- Fluids.
- Silver, water. Gold-touched milk if possible
- Clothes.
- Saffron and pink clothing.
- Ornament.
- Copper, coral.
- Reading.
- Religious, Lovesome, Bravery, Sports books
- Entertaining
- 20-minute stroll with soft music, devotionals, and prayers.
- Contraindication.

- Spicy food, fried food, alcohol, stale and dry meals, overexercising, and travel.

91

Month 3 (1st Trimester)

At the end of 1st trimester,

Starts to react to stimuli

About 2 inches long, the baby starts to move on its own. Mother, start to feel the top of uterus above the pubic bone. With a fetoscope, the doctor may be able to hear the baby's heartbeat. The baby's sex organs should start to become clearer. Developing a sense of smell makes toxic odour unpleasant. The brain grows quickly. It can hear our mother's heartbeat and voice.

Still small, the tummy has lots of room.

Unborn Baby's (UB) Sensory playground is the womb.

UB stretches his/her arms, smiles, and thumb-suck.

Visible organs

Fingers, brain, closed eyes, nose, cheek, tongue, lips, audible heartbeat.

Happiness and sadness emotions expressed.
Human form appearance of foetus.

Nutrition.

- Highly cooked food.
- Milk-sweets.
- Ghee-honey-coconut chutney.
- Indian Gooseberry pickle, fresh turmeric, seasonal fruits and veggies. Dal.

Fluids.

- Coco-water.
- Fennel, rose petals.
- Poppyseed squash
- Gold-infused milk and water.

Clothes.

- Yellow apparel.

Ornament.

- Gold and sapphire jewellery.

Reading.

- Religious prayers for the well-being of UB,
- Good storybooks,

Entertainment.

- 20 minutes' walk in the open air listening to soft music, chanting devotionals, prayers

Contraindication.

- Avoid hot, dry, stale food.

Month 4 (2nd Trimester)

4.3 to 4.6 inches and 3.5 ounces.

- Mother, feel the uterus 3 inches below the belly button.
- The baby's heart and blood vessels are fully formed, and the eyes can blink.
- Digits and toes have fingerprints.
- Half of UB's size is a head.
- Kicking, peeing, and swallowing are learnt.
- Growing taste buds.

If mom consumes a variety of things, we become less picky eaters.

Nutritional deficiencies
"Foetal Programming" adapt our physiology to support development.

This can lead to obesity, heart disease, and diabetes, according to research.

- Womb size and weight increase.
- Fast cardiac development.
- Development emotionally.
- Develop sweat glands.
- Hearing grows.

- The body is smaller than the head

Nutrition.
- Bitter food

Heart-building nutrients.
- Grapes, almonds, butter, citrus, delicious lime, and seasonal produce.
- Fluids.
- Buttermilk.
- Curd-rice. Gold-infused milk and water
- Soup Mint, ginger, and bottle gourd beet.

Clothes.
- Yellowish red and saffron clothing.

Ornament.
- Ruby-and-gold decorations.

Reading.
- Maharana Pratap, Shivaji, Rani Laxmi, Bai, Sardar Patel, Shakti Prapti mantra.

Entertainment.
- 20 minutes' walk in the open air listening to soft music, chanting devotionals, prayers
- Moon viewing Maalkosh.

Contraindication.

- Frightful sites, stale food, and non-vegetarian meals.

Month 5 (2nd Trimester)

10 ounces, 6 inches long.

Uterus at belly button level.

Baby can yawn, stretch, suck thumb and make faces.

"Quickening" is used when a mother starts to feel baby movements. Mom's muffled voice is becoming clearer. UB is growing rapidly. First hair, fingernails, eyebrows, and eyelashes appear. UB becomes more active and loves exercising our muscles.

As UB moves, the mother will feel it.

If the mother reacts with love, UB learns every action has a reply.

Emotional feelings, brain & liver grow. Excretion from the gut occurs. Taste glands develop, and hearing ability increases. Hand movements present

Nutrition.
- Dishes cooked with rice, milk, ghee, and seasonal fruits and vegetables.
- Gooseberry almonds preserve dates.

- Walnut-grapes. Grapes. Fresh lentils, Srikhand, and sweetened curd.
- Fluids.
- water.
- Gold milk.
- Clothes.
- Wearing white.
- Ornaments.
- Pearls and silver.
- Reading.
- Literature.
- Entertainment.
- Yogasan. Pranayama, walking meditation
- Feed pet animals Cows, dogs, ants, and birds.

Contraindication.
- Poor thinking. No actions against conscience. Be calm.

Month 6 (2nd Trimester)

During this sixth month 1.4 lbs.

Moves or increases pulse upon hearing noises. On hiccup, jerking motion develops.

The fully developed inner ear, infants may detect being upside down in utero.

Brain growth milestone "Cerebral cortex divided into hemispheres".

Eyes open now as they can respond to light despite seeing merely blurs.

Mom should take UB outside now.

Makes rudimentary facial expressions, like a "grin". Eventually, UB learns to converse.

Babies want to show feelings when born.

- New hairline.
- Active Census.
- Sucking begins.

Nutrition.

- Raisins, Nuts
- Rice with curd, unrefined sugar, turmeric, raisins. Chinese asparagus.

Fluids.

- Vegetable soup, cows, milk, water, and gold-treated milk.

Clothes.

- Earthy tone
- Sapphire ornaments, earth-toned garments.
- Literature.
- Indian Calendar, Vedic Maths, Bravery Stories, Prayers
- Entertainment.
- Pranayama, asana, Mind-stimulating treks, games, ragtime Deepak

Contraindication

- Poor thinking. No actions against conscience. Be calm

Month 7 (3rd Trimester)

2lbs 6oz Baby

- Often changes position throughout pregnancy.
  The baby would likely survive if delivered preterm now.
- Discuss preterm labour warning signs with your doctor.
- Register for childbirth classes now.
- Birthing classes cover labour and delivery.
- Newborn care and delivery.
- Starts a sleep-wake schedule.
- Hair is now apparent and milk teeth have emerged.
- When UB hears mom, heartbeat and movement rise.
- UB learns language from outside sounds.
- UB prefers the parents' native language once born.

90% probability of surviving if born now.

Full body and organ development.

- Under skin develops.
- Self-sufficient fit.

- Open-and-close eyelids

Nutrition.
- In moderation, taste all
- Oatmeal. Ghee. Raw sugar. Coriander. Rose petals candy. Porridge. Sukhoi. Green-gram products.
- Bottle gourd halwa, ghee-rice.
- Cashews figs. Pistachios.
- Seasonal products.
- Fluids.
- Gram stock. Coco-water.
- Gold-infused pumpkin, water, and milk.
- Clothes. Red attire.
- Ornament.
- Emerald, mica decorations.
- Reading.
- Bravery accounts. Speeches motivating. Gopal. Shakti prapti stotra
- Entertainment.
- Pranayama. Music, meditation. Holy basil pooja massages.
- Blossoms.
- Contraindication.
- Avoid anger.
- And vindictive.

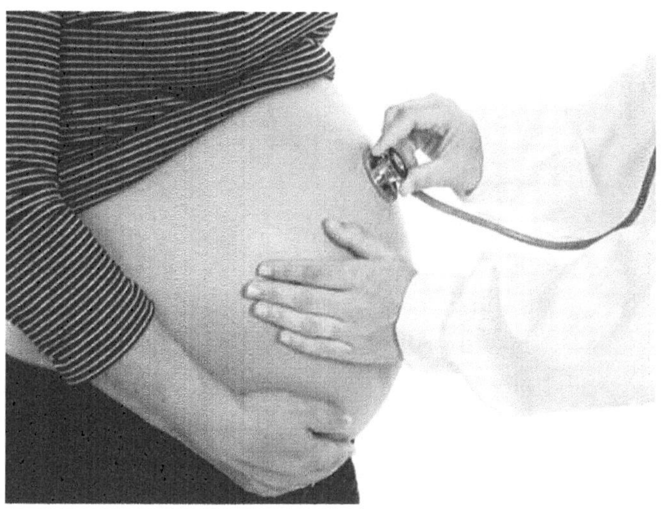

Month 8 (3rd Trimester)

The 4-pound baby is active.

- As fat forms under the baby's skin, wrinkles diminish.
- UB will grow half their birth weight before delivery.
- How to make a foetal movement chart? Get doctors' advice.
- Breastfeed.
- Yellow breast fluid: COLOSTRUM
- Prepare breasts for milk production.
- Visit the doctor every two weeks.
- New-born-like.
- The brain and nervous system are functional.
- UB practises breathing by inhaling amniotic fluid.
- UB spends practically all time sleeping and thinking about the future.
- Most have turned upside down in preparation for birth.
- Bones and skull are flexible to fit through the tunnel's tiny aperture.

- The immune system is young. Internal bodyguards won't be fully effective for months following birth.
- Almost all developments are complete

Nutrition.
- Fenugreek-sweets.
- Goskur Water. Walnut. Rice porridge, Ghevar.
- Other gram. Seasonal Produce.

Fluids.
- Gokshurwater Soup, too.

Clothes.
- White, orange, red.

Ornaments.
Gold.

Reading.
- Religious chants and as specified by the Priests Of Churches or Heads Of Mosque follow them.
- Shrimad Bhagavad-gita.
- Hanuman-chalisa.
- Sunderkand.
- Ganapati mantra.
- Santan stotra.
- Mrityunjaya mantra.

- Kshemkushal

Entertainment.
- Pranayama. Meditation. Walks. Discourses. Positive. Okay.

Contraindication.
- Avoid
- Unpalatable.
- Ice.
- Constipation-causing foods.

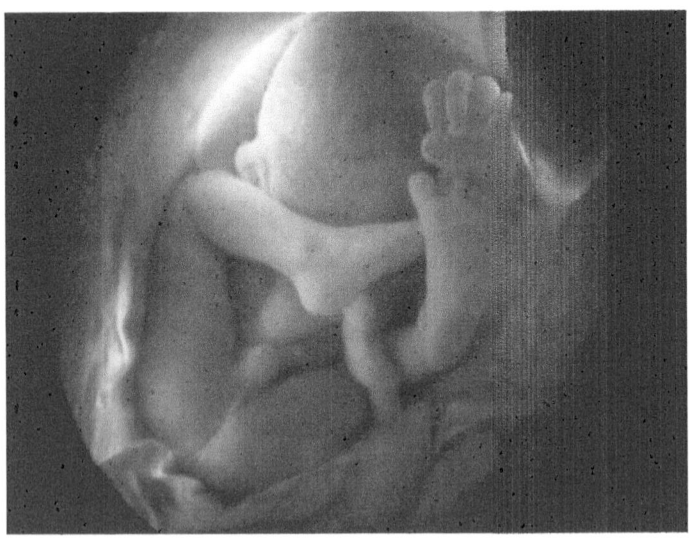

Month 9 (3rd Trimester)

In the last month

- Many factors affect the baby's size.
- Growth pace is as crucial as size.
- A baby at this period is roughly 18.5 inches and 6 pounds.
- Rapid brain growth.
- Nearly-developed lungs
- Now, the head is in the pelvis.
- Born at 37 weeks is a term.
- Born between 37-39 weeks is an early-term baby.
- 39-40 weeks, 41-42 weeks late term.
- UB keeps learning motor skills and kicking.
- Mom laughs, consumes sweets, or drinks iced tea, the UB bounces.
- Mother hopes for a natural delivery that gives UB a stronger immune system for life.
- The riddle of nature vs nurture is well-begun and reveals our character.
- Development of UB is complete

Nutrition.
- Rice-based products.
- Sodium-rich foods.

- Ghee-Walnut Porridge. Cashews. Vegetable greens.
- Souper
- Saffron-milk.
- Gram stock. Soup

Clothes.
- WHITE

Ornaments.
- Golden pearls.

Reading.
- Religious books, as per parents' religion
- Prasav sukha

Entertainment
- Walks, meditation, music, listening.

Contraindication.
- Avoid negativity.
- Angry.
- Fear bad thoughts.

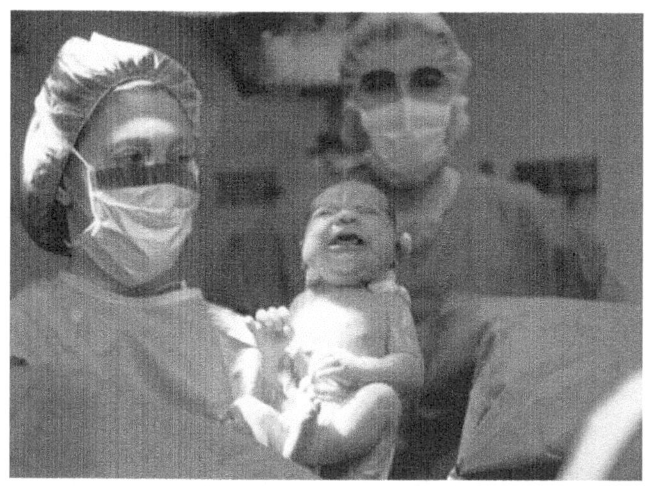

Birth!

Mother's due date marks the end of their 40th week.

Delivery date calculated using the first day of their last period.

Based on this, pregnancy can last between 38 and 42 weeks with a full-term delivery happening around 40 weeks. Post-term pregnancies lasting more than 42 weeks are not really late.

The due date may just not be accurate.

For safety reasons, most babies are delivered by 42 weeks. Doctors may need to induce labour.

Baby's First Cry — Vagitus
The first cry of a baby is called VAGITUS

Vociferous, shrill, and piercing-the first cry of the newborn infant signals that a new and separate life has begun.

Separated from the body of the mother, the newborn cry serves to call for care, support, and protection.

The most joyous moment of a mother's life.

The first cry of the baby is something that signifies his entry into the world.

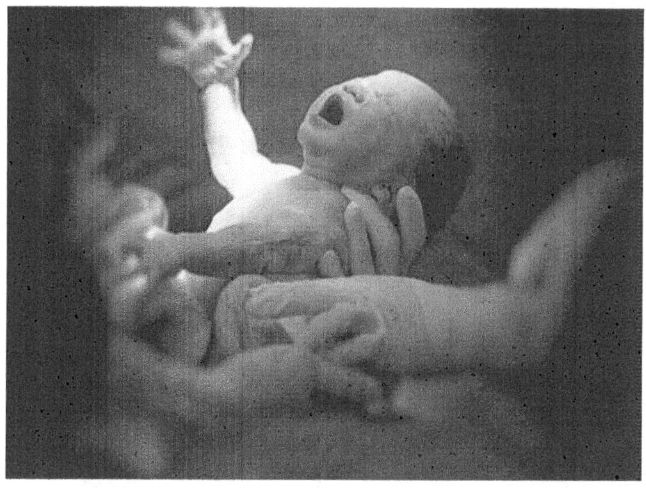

To know More about the Section, Scan the Code

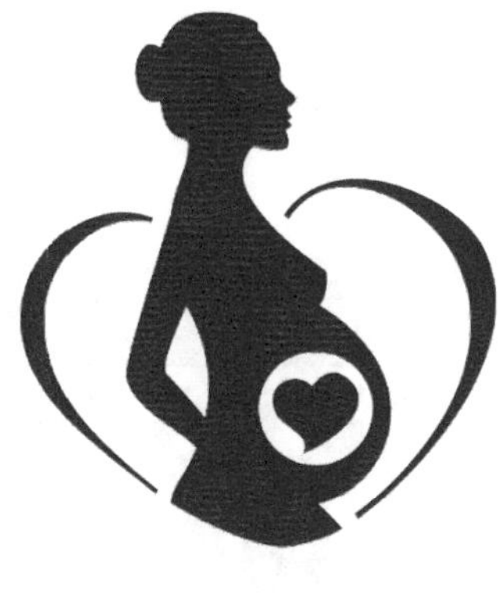

Section 3

Coming Soon!

To know More about the Section, Scan the Code

Notes